22 TIPS TO CHANGE YOUR LIFE

MY TRIP *to a* HEALTHY, ACTIVE

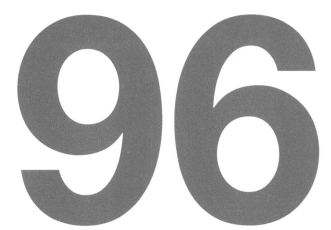

96

BY PHYLLIS SUES

"Perseverance, tenacity and grace mixed with great humor and creativity is what Phylis Sues is all about!"

Marcos Questas

"I have the honor of being her yoga instructor and friend for over ten years. I have been in awe of her since the first day she did Peacock Pose, one of the most challenging poses in yoga. Her passion for life is unmatched even for people a quarter her age. I can only hope to live that long and with such joy."

Anthony Benanati

Photography by Adam Sheridan-Taylor,
(unless otherwise noted).

Book layout by Paul Manchester
FugitiveColors.com

These fitness exercises have been useful for Phyllis Sues.
Your circumstances may vary and you should first consult your
medical professional to see if these exercises might be right for you.

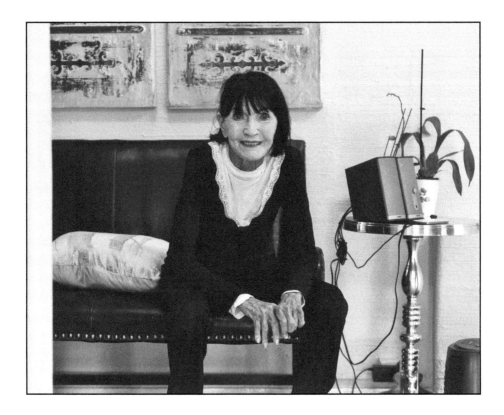

I'm driven to tell this story and write this book.

My amazing journey started on my 18th birthday when I began living, working, and dancing on Broadway. Five musicals: *Oklahoma, Brigadoon, Bloomer Girl, High Button Shoes,* and *Kismet.* After those lucrative and formative years, I performed with Alan Sues doing comedy at *Le Reuben Bleu* – a fashionable nightclub in New York, in addition to taking our act to many other venues.

At age 50, I opened my own studio and successful fashion business for twenty-two years. After which I produced and created two CDs. *Scenes Of Passion* – twelve songs for which I wrote lyrics and music, followed by *Tango Insomnia* which had six tangos. Both can be found on *Amazon* and *iTunes.* Not to be stopped, I returned to the world of dance and performed Argentine Tango at age 92 which went viral internationally on *YouTube.*

At 85 I stepped into my first yoga class. All during this time I was busy writing forty blogs for *The Huffington Post.* I danced and was interviewed on the *The Queen Latifah Show,* and did headstands with Katie Couric.

For at least ten years, I have been inspiring thousands of men and women of all ages to follow my tips. So follow my tips. I know the method. It takes desire, followed by action, and above all the recognition and acceptance of challenge. The magic words are OPEN UP and say *"Good Morning, Good Morning I Love This Day".* You can be a winner. It's not about looking young, it's about feeling better, liking what you do, and above all liking yourself and who you are. Important but not so simple.

This book is composed of some yoga poses with photos, some exercises I've developed, plus my philosophy of the partnership of body and mind – all of which **if followed** will change your life.

Sincerely,
Phyllis Sues

Ways to Live – Not Just Exist

Time
Take advantage of time
Enjoy time of itself
Enjoy time with yourself
Enjoy time to know yourself
Enjoy time to like yourself

Simplify your life.

Hard to achieve, beautiful to perceive, and amazing to own.

Living beyond 90 can be a rich and rewarding experience. You need to listen to the silence and realize the importance of space between thoughts, words, and movements.

You may move slower but in a nurturing way. Create an adventure, one that fits your parameters. Be adventurous, daring, childlike.

It's your right, your time, and no guilt. You own the right to be you. If not now, when? It's time.

The word *possible* is a key word to longevity. **You will work harder for the result if you think it's possible.** If it's possible, if it's credible, then it's doable.

There's significance in the word difference. Want the difference, desire it. Know the difference is there. If you know it the difference will be there. Take action and you will make the difference.

Your life is worth it.

At this time in your life, you have the privilege of enjoying freedom. Mental, physical and emotional. Fatigue can be a joy if you're doing something you like.

I love practicing yoga. The fatigue that comes after a yoga class is my reward. It can be yours at any age. There is no excuse not to practice yoga. It comes at all levels.

Beyond 90 is the time to let go.
Time to forgive.
Time to know and like yourself.
Time to have fun, no strings attached, no guilt.
Give yourself and body the life it never had.
Accept the challenges and make choices.
Now you're living.
The journey is just beginning.

Go beyond your comfort zone. That takes determination, dedication and effort.

Sitting in a chair won't cut it. It's a matter of pushing yourself that extra inch.

You have been given an amazing instrument. It's your responsibility to give it an amazing life.

You want to live, not just exist.
There is a difference.
Now is the time to make that difference.
You and your body are a team.
Have fun together.
It's never too late!

It's never too late to do the gym.
Never too late to run and swim.
Never too late to appreciate.
Always too late to vacillate.
Don't hesitate just generate.
So recreate and motivate.
What are you waiting for?
Eating and sleeping?
There must be something more?

You have to start somewhere.
Why not here and now.
Try this basic exercise.
Get up out of a chair 10 times in succession.
Hands on your hips.
Don't forget to breathe.
Oh, well, just a thought.

Say, *"Good morning, good morning I love this day."* Just this line can change the way you feel about yourself and this day. Each day is an awakening and it's a new journey every day.

You will never live to be 100 unless you realize the importance of freedom. Physical and mental. Living is a challenging exercise and it takes desire, inspiration, and action to achieve a healthy and creative life at whatever age. Don't put the brakes on just because you're more than 90. That's just the time to accelerate.

Again.
It's never too late to do the gym.
It's never too late to run and swim.
So what are you waiting for?
Eating and sleeping?
There must be something more?

Being 20 is not better than being 90+, it's just different. I'm more aware of being here, more appreciative of being alive. More compassionate. More patient. And more cognizant of loving what I do. Yes, it's different and better.

Tango with my teacher, Marcos Questas.

That being said, if you give your body an amazing life then 90+ will be better.

Do something that stimulates your body.
Yoga stimulates and relaxes both body and mind.
Yoga is a reason to wake up each morning.

Solving problems is easier.
Your life is simplified.

Life is not easy
but it sure beats not being here at all.
Take a day at a time.
It's living one by one.
"Retire" you just gave up!
Take on a new project
something that stimulates both mind and body.
Ballroom dancing
Tango
Foreign language
Ceramics
Painting

I could go on and on, there is no limit.
Reinvention is the perfect step forward.

I know that better is better than not good enough. Not good enough stops the engine. Better means there's another chance. Another step on the ladder.

To introduce something new in your life you need to open your eyes, your ears, and your mind. Something new in your life is a wire you can grab hold of at any age.

So lighten up, experiment, have fun. You might surprise yourself.

There is a reward for every minute of physical practice and that reward is feeling your best possible best. It's a full time job.

Let's not try it, let's do it. If you take that extra step today, tomorrow you'll love yourself.

It's the process of learning that makes living worth living at any age. When you're in the process of what you chose to do you're in the process of living. So grab hold of the wire and fly.

It's never ever too late.

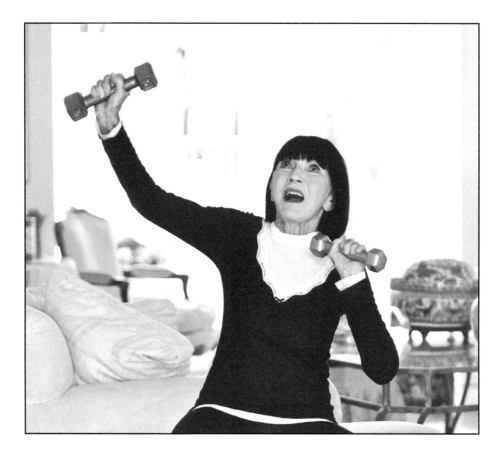

Tip #1 In Gear

I feel I have the right to encourage you to use your body and mind. You need your mind to put your body in drive and your body to take action.

This trio is:

Inspire, Desire, Action.

This trio works.

I got to 96 for a good reason.

Dedication to the process of living, effort, desire, no fear. The love of challenge, and above all - *It's never ever too late.*

That challenge started at age 14 and a ballet lesson with the famous George Balanchine. That lesson put me in gear for the rest of my life.

Together you and I can start the motor. And you and your body and mind will say "I can do it."

IT'S NEVER EVER TOO LATE!

This book is not just my journey to age 96, but my desire to inspire and give you a real and healthy life.

We can do it together.

Tip #2 Best Friend

Your body is your best friend, you are partners. You have to respect, honor, and love this miraculous piece of machinery the universe has given you. You were born to move with wonderful oiled joints and muscles, and everything you could possibly need to show the world how beautiful you are.

I'll help, but you have to accept the challenge, and **the challenge is *planned activity.*** Do you want a better physical life? Then let's start when the sun shines or when the first rays of daylight spread the sky with these words, *"Good Morning, Good Morning I love this day."*

I've been saying, *"Good Morning, Good Morning I love this day"* for most of my life. Even for each audition and there were many. Five hit Broadway shows, four careers with one thought: I can do it. I talked and pushed my body to the limit.

It was always one word: *I'm ready* (well two words). The challenges have always been waiting out there, and I've always been ready. *Now, it's your turn to be ready.*

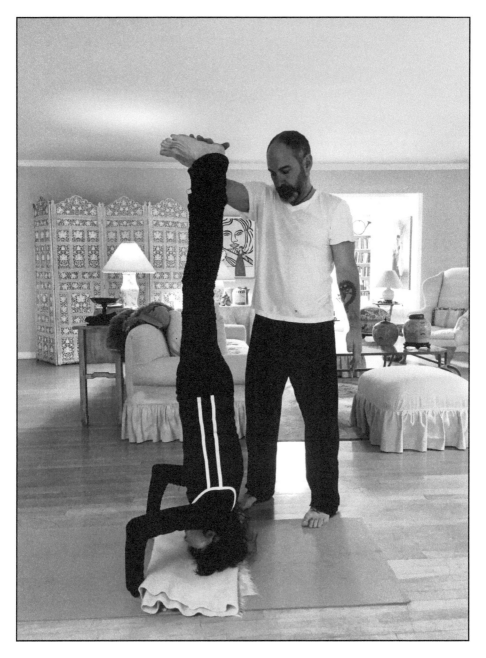

With Anthony Benenati,
my best friend and yoga mentor.

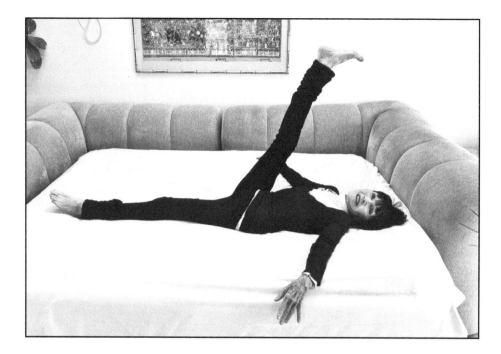

TIP #3 Leg Raises - Straight

You can begin on your bed and start with simple **stretches - repeat this leg motion raising each leg waist level five times. Rhythmically. No resting.** Just repeat this with the other leg.

You can do it. Don't forget to breathe.

The magical word is *dedication.* The guy on a mat next to me said it would take me ten years to do a handstand. Well, it's ten years and I still cannot do a handstand. But I wont give up.

This is your mantra: *Never Give Up.*

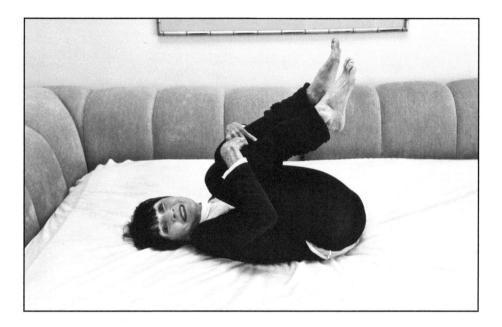

TIP #4 Leg Raises Bent to Chest

We're still on the bed, but **now we're raising both legs together, but with bent knees. Keeping legs bent, touch your chest with your knees.** You'll feel a nice stretch in your back.

You can do it. Now just hold that position for the count of twenty.

WOW, I like that.

You can do it. You did it!

It's the gym. It's yoga. It's the walk, the jog, the jump rope. I can think of ten things to make a difference in your life. But you have to want to do it and you have to do it.

No would, could, should – just do it.

Here's what I sing when I wake up just to make sure I'm completely here and ready for this day.

> *In the morning and at night,*
> *all day long it's a delight.*
> *Doing stretches to my song –*
> *killer handstands two minutes long,*
> *twenty squats, jumping rope,*
> *It's my rite to live this life.*

Below is a warm up for the real thing, which you will find in chapter 16. Do this pose on both right and left sides.

Doing the real thing is a difficult balancing act.

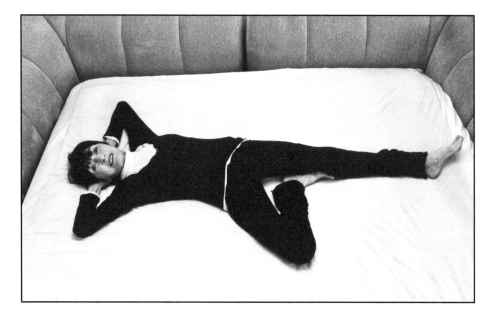

Tip #5 Opening Doors

Life is a series of numbers.

As the numbers grow, so does life, and as life grows we must accept each number as a challenge. You will hear me repeat the word challenge many times. There's a reason. **Repetition is a builder of strength, memory, even joy.**

When you go to the gym, you repeat the exercises. In yoga, we repeat the poses. *Practice involves repetition.*

Life is a series of numbers. As the numbers grow, so does life. And as life grows, we must accept each number as a challenge and a door. The word challenge and the acceptance of each challenge is how and why we become who we are. Seeing, accepting, and facing each challenge is your way of living a healthy life both physically and mentally.

Now the numbers are endless. And opening the door to each challenge is the best choice you have.

Hello Tip #6 Uttanasana

Uttanasana (forward bending)

I have to admit there will be days when you feel good about yourself. You may even like yourself. And then there will be days where you feel like shit. I'm 96. I'm privileged with profanities. So you can't move? You just want to lie in bed? So be it. Then the days when you feel great make up for the shitty days.

Uttanasana is the simplest looking and the most difficult to do with perfection. It takes long and limber leg muscles. With that said, it's probably the most practiced in yoga class. But we're going to give it a go. I like doing better than try. **Try means maybe, do means DO.**

Stand on both straight legs, now reach for the floor – touching the floor with both hands. If not possible to touch the floor, place some books to make it possible to touch the books. Remain in this pose touching the floor or books for

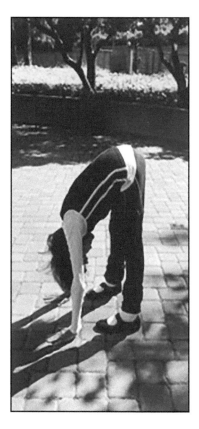

thirty seconds. Now stand up straight with arms overhead and reach for the sky. Do this complete pose reaching the floor then reaching the sky at least five times. This is great for stamina – core and legs. Don't give up on this. It's your ticket to strength. It's a combination of the most important, the simplest looking, but the most difficult to master.

Do this every morning when you sing, *Good Morning I love this day.* This is really good after you've done your stretches on the bed. Your body needs those stretches, cries for them. Don't cheat. Do them if not for me for you. Your body is sending you a message, LISTEN.

I'm going to slip in and out of yoga poses which you can't beat, and my own invented poses and exercises. They don't call yoga exercise, they call it practice. I call mine *living in challenge.*

Tip #7 The Winner - Wall Squat

Living is one helluva profession. I should know I've been at it for 96 years.

When you become a living part of this universe your primal instinct tells you to open your lungs and say, HELLO AND MOVE. Your education has just begun and the moment of learning how to move.

So what happened between then and now?

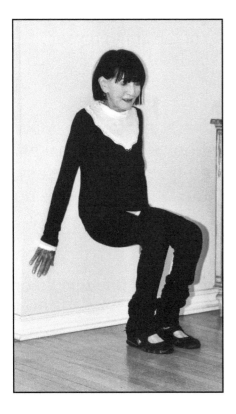

This is the first step into the profession of living. The staring into the face of challenge. And if we're smart enough to deal with the challenge, then the profession of living is no longer a marathon – it's the winning ticket.

So here we go with the winning ticket.

It's called **The Wall Squat** - leaning against a wall, drop your body into a chair position (see photo).

Remain in this position for at least 1 minute.

Your body and legs should be in an L shape and the deeper you drop your body the better the result. This takes strength in every part of your body, but mainly in your thighs and your butt. Push hard against the wall. You can do it. *This is a building pose.*

Breathe and count. Count out loud. Counting out loud keeps you on target. **For all these exercises count out loud.** You'll find counting out loud, or even just simply counting quietly becomes a habit so habitual you begin to wonder. Counting two minutes is not only good for Wall Squat but a great sleep aid.

I find myself counting to myself for absolutely no reason. Maybe it takes the place of talking to myself.

But back to the Wall Squat.

Yes I know your thighs are burning and you say WOW this is pain, but don't you give up! Hold one minute. You're not going to die – not yet. I know it's not easy. Even I feel pain holding two minutes. I refuse to give up to less than two minutes no matter how much my thighs are killing me.

So if I can do two minutes, you can do one minute or maybe forty-five seconds. I'm giving you a break.

I want you to have fun doing this program. If fun enters into it then you will do it. Right!!

If not for you, then for me because I'm watching.

Let's take one minute break and go back to the subtitle do you want *22 Tips That Can Change Your Life*? We're only up to #7, so maybe we, you and I, haven't changed your life yet. There are a few miles ahead.

Together we're going to think about muscles and celebrate their very existence, and all the amazing things we will do for strength, power and energy. It's possible and doable.

If your life is better, my life is better.

So here comes #8.

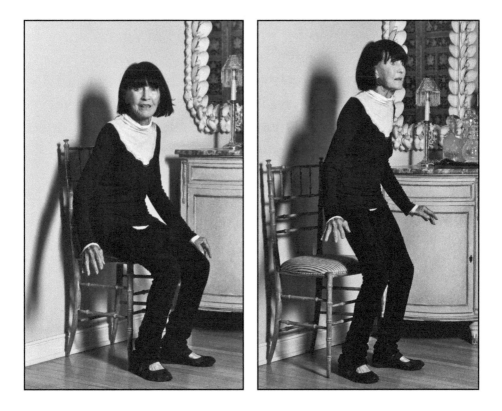

TIP #8 CHAIR

This exercise sounds easy. You start sitting in a chair. Wood or iron is a good choice. **You are going to rise up to standing position with absolutely no assistance from hands or arms -** no leaning forward as you rise and sit. It's simply you and your own body strength. Done correctly it's not easy. It takes core strength.

Repeat this five times I really want you to get to ten times. Breathing all the time. Remember that word - **breathe** - it's your gift of life.

Did I hear something that sounds like "I don't have time?" You just stopped progress and lost a piece of your life.

We live by the word time
and we take time to live.
We take time to breathe.
Time to sleep.
Time to think.

Time between thoughts.
Time between words.
And most of all time to be inspired and
feel better doing these 22 tips.
If you feel better, I'll feel better.
So let's work together.
It's worth the time.

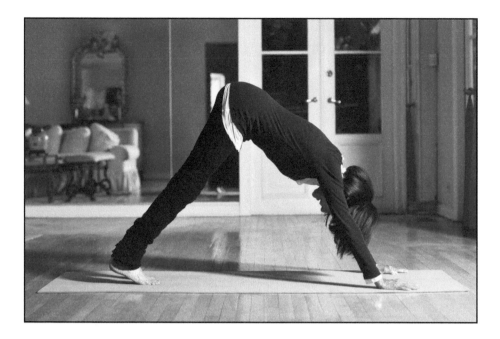

Tip #9 Down Dog

Next is a basic yoga pose, **Down Dog.**

It's not difficult.

There are some yoga poses you can't beat or improve upon and this is one of them. The results are tremendous.

You need to settle in this pose for one minute. It happens to be a cure-all for many things. Number one, it strengthens the entire body. It has been known to cure stomach aches, head aches, and even diarrhea. I know from personal experience.

Now just take a minute and think about what it's like to simply be alive. You never compliment this amazing machine.

Take a second and look at your feet. How many millions of miles in a lifetime have they carried you, walking, running, jumping, running marathons, how about just standing in line?

My God, speak to them, massage them and love them. Whose fault is their injury? Most injuries are a result of not being present or just careless. Sometimes moving too fast. Thinking about what you forgot to do, but definitely not what you were doing. I love the word DO. It replaces SHOULD, WOULD, and COULD, which inevitably means not done.

Your body is a Stradivarius. For it to respond with a beautiful tone, you have to love it and practice on it every day. My body is my Stradivarius. I say thanks every waking and sleeping moment for the amazing gift my mother gave birth to. Even at birth I had such energy, curiosity, and elasticity. The world was a wonderland, a treasure, and it belonged to me.

I don't do the things that I do because I think I *should* do them. I jump rope four minutes every day because it feels so good to jump rope. I practice yoga because it makes me feel better, and I practice tango because I'm in love with the dance form and the music. All this produces incredible joy and a creative and healthy life and body.

So if you go to the gym because you feel you must go to the gym, instead of *I love all the exercises, and those exercises give me and my body the breath of life.* What more can one ask?

It's basically all about loving what you do and why you do it.

The reason you don't move?
You get in the way.
You were born to move.
Give your beautiful instrument a break.
Love it, teach it, train it.
Allow the energy it owns to have a life.

"I can't do that because..."

The word *because* is a killer and does nothing to correct the problem.

"because I'm too old"

"because I have arthritis"

"because I have osteoporosis"

Almost all can be improved with activity. Arthritis responds to activity. I know because my body is full of arthritis. Shoulders, knees, feet, hands.

I will not allow arthritis to take over my life.

The only solution is major activity.

And the best way to practice major activity is yoga with a huge Y. Take the first step with a yoga class. Your body will be hooked. You may not be, but your body is talking.

So listen. Your Stradivarius is so expensive there is no number on its value. Only you know it's value. So keep it well tuned. The music it will produce will be beautiful, powerful, and rewarding. **You have been given this incredible instrument - your first and only instrument.**

Love it, and give it the life it deserves.

What a Gift WOW !!!!!!

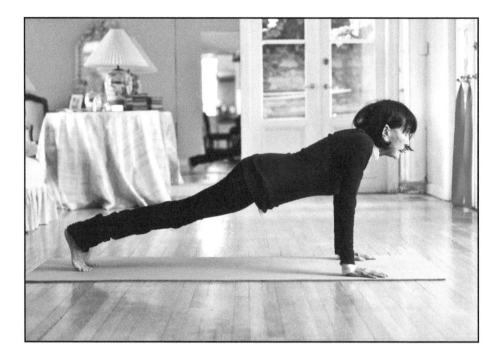

Tip #10 Plank

It's a winner and its called **Plank.**

Do this pose one minute.

It looks so easy and it's so difficult, but do not skip this pose. **Your body is suspended above the floor by your hands and feet.** It takes strength and it builds strength. This will put pressure on both hands, arms and shoulders. Can't tell you how important this pose is.

When I do Plank for three minutes my entire body is shaking. You can see the position of the body is completely straight just like a plank. Do not allow your body to collapse. Plank is a very popular yoga pose, but not many can achieve one minute. I want to show them you can do Plank two minutes. If you can hold this pose one minute BRAVO. May take a little time to hold two minutes.

Keep trying don't give up.
Do it Do it Do it.
It's worth it, I promise.

Aging, can be exciting, creative, active, and even daring. But (and it's a huge but), it's not easy to own this. It's work, desire, and challenging, And most of all loving what you do.

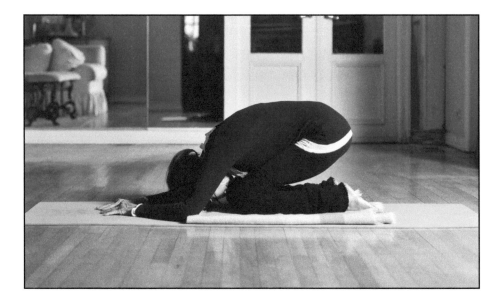

Tip #11 Child Pose

This pose is a delicious way in which to move after Plank. **Child Pose takes you into a quiet and a very private world. One becomes centered and calm.**

It's a place in which time is of the essence. A time to enjoy and feel the universe. It's a place to be completely present. You will welcome this pose after Plank.

The longer you're in Plank, the better Child Pose feels. In Child Pose, I own myself. I'm in a private world.

Awakening The Seed Of Creativity

What is the motivation for living?
What is the motivation for getting out of that bed?
What is the motivation for looking good?

What is the motivation for feeling good?
What is the motivation to accept each challenge?

These questions plague the universe.

But there is a way I'm motivated, because I cannot face the possibility that my body and mind will be any less tomorrow than it is today. And I have pride, energy, and endless desire to be better not just tomorrow, but every day.

I only have me, and that's all each one of us has. No one is going to do it for you. You and you alone are the engine.

To be inspired is a dead end unless you do something about it. To be inspired is one thing, To do something about it is another thing entirely.

And having desire goes nowhere unless you take action. **Inspiration, desire, and action. All three together make a life worth living.**

Take a deep breath and enjoy the silence that comes with deep breathing in the Child Pose and it's possible you may discover a seed of creativity hidden away. It needs to be awakened.

Tip #12 FEET

We are back on the bed, but now we are going to work with your feet. As we grow, our feet do nasty tricks. Like arthritis and neuropathy. I have both. And if you've never had either, lucky you. But even if you are one of the lucky ones, these next exercises will insure you of healthy feet and also make them feel good.

Now lean over and touch your feet if you are limber, if not bend both knees or just one knee at a time. You use both hands and both feet putting your fingers on your right hand between each toe on your right foot, and fingers on left hand between the toes on the left foot.

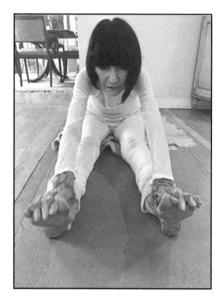

Remain in this position for forty-five seconds.

My toes and feet love this one - and this next one too. Again, right hand on right foot left hand on left foot. Now wrap each hand around all toes then bend the toes forward hold for forty-five seconds. Then do the same thing but bend the toes toward you.

I've been dancing tango in three inch heels for ten years with no pain – *if I can, you can.* **But I do these foot exercises every day.**

Ninety percent of people walking the earth are either overweight, bent over with curvature of the spine, and – lets not talk about feet. Help is needed!

My audience is inspired but that doesn't mean they do anything to change their physical situation. There is help out there. Yoga, Pilates, the gym, and of course ME.

Stick with me. I promise results.

I admit physical activity can produce fatigue, even pain but there is pleasure from both - **no pain, no gain.**

Viva La Difference

*Do you realize how incredible you are
to have gotten this far?
You are only as old as you think you are.
Now, start a new page.
Enjoy the thought of what is possible.
Thinking you can, you will
go for the reality. Clean up your act.
Exercise more than you think you should.
Don't allow fatigue to get in your way.
Take advantage of time.
Enjoy time with yourself.
Enjoy time to know yourself.*

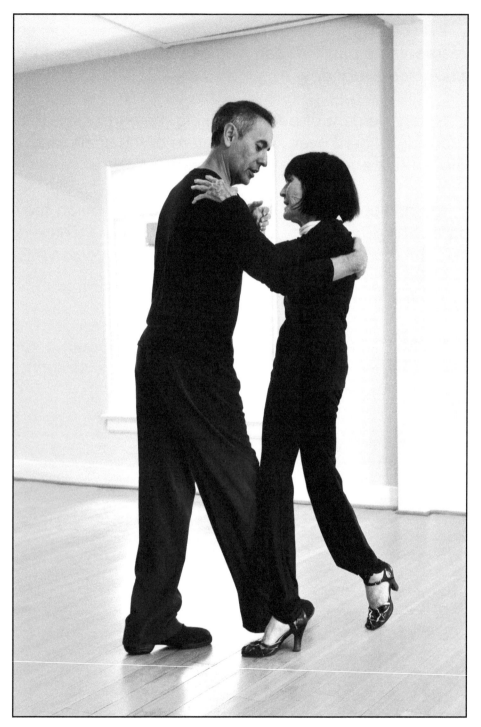

Tango with my teacher, Marcos Questas, who taught me to follow.

And above all,
enjoy time to like yourself.
No looking or living ahead.
The secret is now, not yesterday, or tomorrow,
simply NOW.
Simplify your life.
Hard to achieve, but beautiful to perceive,
and amazing to own.

Living can be a rich and rewarding experience.
It takes two kinds of energy, mental and physical.
Be adventuresome, daring, and childlike.
It's your prerogative, your right and your time.
The difference is not the number.
The number is a devious device.
It's not how much time I have.
It's how much better time I will have.
Wake up and live,
or sit in that chair and do nothing.
Enjoy the thought of what's possible
then go for the reality.
Thinking you will, you will invent and simplify.
It's not the number. No need to slow down.
The need is to accelerate.
Put your foot on the pedal and go for it.

So the difference is the possible.
The credible and yes the doable.
Not only does it sound good, it is good.
Barbra Streisand uses space between lyrics.
When you use space,
you become aware of silence,
and with silence comes knowledge.

Using time and space to it's fullest can lead to a creative and rich life.

Simplification will create space. It's not a secret. So want the difference, desire it, know that it's there. Take action and you will make the difference, your life is worth it.

The Difference Between 96 and 20

The difference between 96 and 20? Right away, you'll throw up your hands and not want to deal with that subject.

But take a moment and listen.
At 96 I have wisdom.
That word at 20 is not even known.
At 96, I pretty much know who I am.
At 20, I hadn't a clue.
At 96, I've faced the bumps large and small,
lost some, won some.
At 20, those bumps are just showing up
for better or worse.
At 96, you've won or lost,
but it's happened.
At 20, you are probably not yet the winner
and wondering when and if you'll hold the trophy.
At 96, I have complete freedom
to do what I want to do,
*to think **how** I want to think,*
*and **what** I want to think,*
and above all to make decisions.
At 20, all these pieces of freedom are questionable.
Yes, you are right.
I speak for myself, and
you at whatever age must learn to do the same.
It's living without fear.

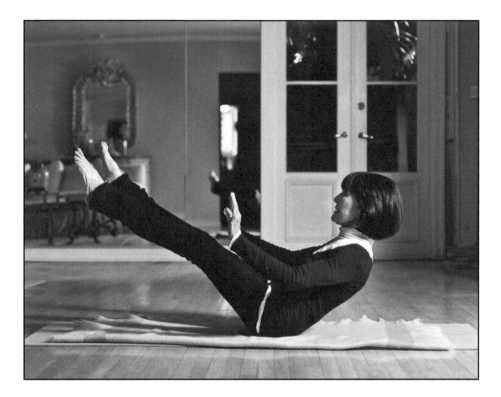

Tip #13 Boat

If you are one of the lucky ones with a gorgeous flat tummy, then this tip is only for you to maintain that gorgeous, flat tummy. All my other readers interested in bikinis and strappy dresses should listen and check out the **Boat.**

Lying flat on your back on the floor or mat, raise your legs to a nearly half way position. And raise your torso to the same nearly half way position, so you are in the same pose as the photo.

Now hold that pose for eight slow counts. Then lower both legs and torso to the floor. Now repeat this exercise the exact same way, holding eight counts each time.

Maybe you won't have that gorgeous flat tummy in one week, but if you are a good girl and repeat this each day for two weeks, you might see and feel something different happening.

Just one other small suggestion. How about the diet? Didn't mean to introduce this ugly word, but it's a thought that always needs tackling. I'm sure you don't absolutely adore this suggestion, but just between you and me, give it a try. No I didn't mean that. I mean give it a do. **Do is the magic word.**

And out comes the bikini.

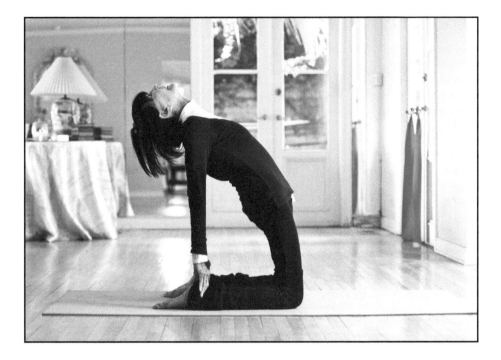

Tip #14 Camel

Did you ever see a camel on his knees, or I should say did you ever see a camel? Either way, right now, you will be a camel on your knees looking up at the beautiful sky. **Leaning back in a back bend, reach with your hands and touch your ankles. You're now in a semi back bend.**

It's not so easy, but it's a great stretch. Bend as far as you can.

This will put lots of pressure on your thighs at the same time giving your back a real stretch. Hold this position for thirty seconds.

If you can hold it for one minute, you're giving your back a real test, and giving yourself something special.

I can do it.

It's all about self (numero uno), and right now I want you (numero uno) to feel good about *yourself.*

I'm completely cognizant of the fact that doing an exercise upon waking to this glorious day and your life is not always exactly what you want to do.

I also have these mornings. But I also know this body at 96 needs enormous help to simply maintain, maybe not even get better because muscles age as does the mind, so it's my job and now your job to put yourself in drive.

And this performance takes will power and drive, but gives results. If I can do it, *you can do it.*

This is not a joke, this is fact.

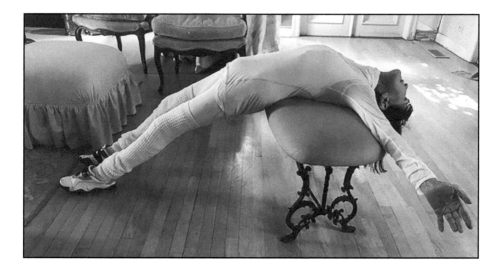

Tip #15 Comfort Zone

This is one without fear or pain. This challenge is what I call comfort.

So find a piece of furniture. You will need something like a bench so you can lie over it not on your stomach but on your back legs stretched out straight, and arms stretched out to either side of your shoulders. For me this pose eases all pain in the back. I can rest in this pose for at least one or two minutes.

I have stenosis of the spine - deterioration of certain discs. So this opens them up. *So after remaining in this pose my whole torso speaks in pluses. This outshines an epidural shot.*

My living room has become my gym and I have a large dog who encourages me.

Delicate Balance

Now that your body has taken a rest, let's try something more taxing. It's so simple – the word that is, **Balance.**

I don't remember balance ever being a factor until the number 85 rolled around and captured my attention. I was just starting to learn tango, and hand in hand with that came yoga. Both of which cannot be achieved without good balance plus quite a few other things. Like for instance: energy, strength, concentration, passion, and simplicity.

But balance spoke to me and demanded to be heard, so I've been working on balance for eight years. And it just occurred me, balance isn't achieved physically without the mentality working in unison. These two talented pieces of machinery are a major part of your instrument.

Another way of creating this miracle is the word presence or being aware - which takes a great deal of concentration. It's not unlike meditation. **We are constantly losing that awareness and then we lose our balance.**

To my complete astonishment the solution was staring me in my face. It's a duet between mind and body, and it's easy to slip in and out of this duet and presence.

It's simplistic, but simplicity is the most difficult to achieve and the most surprisingly beautiful to perceive.

At a certain time in our life in this universe, one never

knows the exact time, it just happens and we start to lose our balance.

The medical profession has all sorts of reasons but no solutions. I can do a million exercises and still not find balance. But the minute I conscientiously listen to my mind working with my body there comes a small degree of balance, and I have discovered several very basic practices.

And here they are:
1. Bare feet, stand straight, feet together, hands at your side.
2. Close your eyes for thirty seconds.
3. Same position, rise up on balls of your feet for thirty seconds with your eyes open.
4. If you succeed with #3, do it with your eyes closed.

(I didn't say TRY, I said DO. There is one more.)

5. Same posture standing on right leg, raise left leg just a few inches from off the floor.
6. Now standing on left leg, raise right leg a few inches off the floor.

Tie your physicality and your mentality in a strong knot. They need to live and work together.

Every step I take, I send a message to my muscles that support and create my balance. When I do that, I feel secure on my feet and immediately find balance.

The balancing exercises are a great gift, as is jump rope. I find I can't give up jump rope entirely even though I'm advised to lay off. I love it, my heart loves it, my feet, my ankles, my knees, my arms, and shoulders love it. Maybe my spine is not so crazy about it, but it's outnumbered.

Balance is just as much mental as it is physical. I'm not just theorizing about this process, it's something quite real. This practice... and it is *a practice.*

My mind and my body are working together. They are having a conversation and it goes like this:

> *Tighten your butt muscles*
> *Pull in your core*
> *Tighten your thighs*
> *Shoulders back*
> *Feel your ankles*
> *Even your toes*

Now your entire body and mind will take notice.

You will feel strength and at the same time a softness. In a word, CALM.

I've been dancing tango seven years and I see this feeling in professional tango dancers, and until now I've never been able to feel it in myself. You'll know it and you'll feel it when you've attained it. Only then are you aware and totally present. I don't have this amazing feeling one hundred percent, but now that I know what the sensation feels like I will never give it up.

I can still remember at age eighteen standing on point in my little pink toe shoes in arabesque for thirty seconds – that's called balance..

Now simply doing a perfect tango walk front and back takes all my strength. When done well it looks like total simplicity. Simplicity is so difficult to achieve and so beautiful to perceive.

Life is a balancing act and every thing that makes it balanced is up to us. It's taken me 96 years to understand and reckon with, and act upon this new found knowledge. It's not magical. It's acceptance, concentration, and lots of work. All in that order.

I've been cooperating with this astonishing universe 96 years.

My mission from now on is to achieve perfect balance and help you to do the same.

You've just been doing balancing exercises and now comes the perfect way to achieve what you just practiced.

That is if you did.

Lets go for a real balancing act – Tree Pose.

Tip #16 Tree Pose (Standing)

You've already done this pose, but on the bed. That was a piece of cake. **Now you are going to do it standing on your left leg, then your right leg.**

I like to start on my left leg, because my right leg and foot touching the inside of my left knee sounds physically impossible, but check out the photo! It's not physically impossible, so balance on your left leg. So sorry to say this, but for me it's like going to Mars. Now reverse and balance on your right leg with your left foot touching the inside of your right knee. If you're now not totally confused, maybe I should start all over again. Or maybe you should just take a look at the photo.

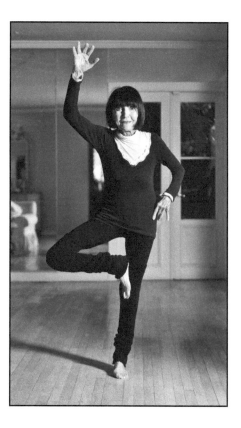

96 years of physical training and my balance is not one hundred percent, so go figure. Some people no matter what age can stand on one leg and balance for hours.

Not my good fortune. Either you have good balance or you don't.

But go for it. You might just be one of the lucky ones. Yet, I can do splits on both sides. We are all so very unique - that's the good news.

Tree Pose is just gorgeous when one is balancing and it takes strength both physical and mental to accomplish this.

Yes, lots easier on the bed right?

I'm challenging you and that's a word to be dealt with.

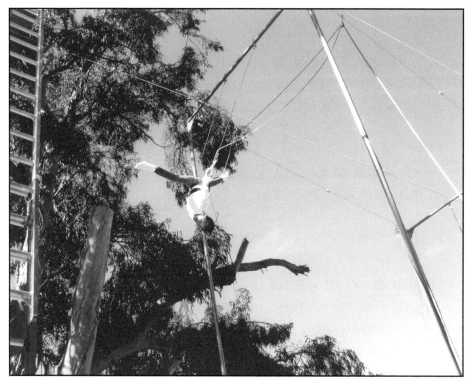

On the trapeze in my 80s (photo taken by my step-son, Charles)

Tip #17 Challenge

We all have this energy, strength and drive. For years it can be hidden deep inside and then one day something clicks. It's like an embryo that awakens. It's that magical combo of mind and body working together.

So I'm asking you to take the challenge. Go for it.

When daylight spreads its wings, its your turn to take off with desire and action. Face the challenge!

Let's not talk about *haven't got time* again.

The process of change is not always speedy. It takes time. It takes dedication, desire, and the belief that it's possible, and above all the ability to accept the challenge. That's asking a lot I know.

Even at 96, I'm still learning, practicing, and testing my body. No matter how tired I am, or even sick, I hate to even mention that word sick. I'm rarely sick.

I admit I'm driven by desire. That's the formula.

Desire is so powerful that you are propelled as if by a canon. Desire is the driving force, but action is the result. Working and accomplishing something mental and physical makes my day worth living. Suddenly there is a break-through, another step on the ladder. I don't give up.

The sun and the moon are out there for everyone.
The journey is worth it.
There is a way to beat the clock.
Stay fit, enjoy the journey.
Accept the challenge and go for it.
Say "Good Morning" and look for the challenge.

When I was 75, I took an extension course at UCLA to learn Italian. If you don't train the body it withers. If you don't train the mind, you lose it. After learning Italian, I tackled French and wrote music and lyrics to my first song *Free Fall,* which was inspired by flying on the trapeze. A CD followed with twelve songs – *Scenes Of Passion* and then six tangos – *Tango Insomnia.*

I now write short songs daily about things I do. That amuses my dog. Fear is a killer of creativity. Desire dispels fear. Fear is not a word in my vocabulary, nor is *should, would,* or *could.*

I became really creative when I opened my fashion business and designed a successful line of women's sportswear. At the end of 22 years it was time to move on. And with a gift of a Steinway Grand piano, I closed my studio and fell headlong into music. This amazing journey is still traveling.

If every part of you is inactive, it causes mental and physical depression, and creativity dies.

TRAPEZE

did I know it was going to be like this
did I know it was going to be such bliss
doing yoga
dancing tango
flying on a trapeze
we practiced outdoors
under the trees
did I know this could be me in a split
somersault off the bar land on my knees
do a catch and not miss

oh my, did I know life could be like this
the best part of did I know
I didn't know
the best part of tomorrow
is
I don't know

do you?

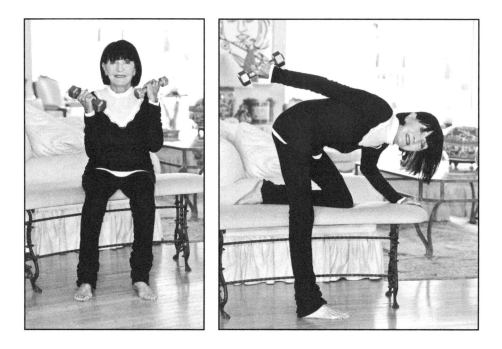

Tip #18 Weights: A Zinger

What has happened to my arms? I have all those neat strappy dresses just hanging in my closet, but I need help.

Well, here I am, your five pound weights. **You think weights are strictly gym equipment, but you're wrong. Haha! You can do weights on a plane, in your bedroom, kitchen or living room.** There is no space needed. For biceps and triceps you just need your desire and plenty of action.

I'm giving you a break with only five pound weights to start for both biceps and triceps. **Put one weight in each hand. Stand up with both arms at your side. Raise the weights to your shoulder with arms bent keeping**

elbows at waist. Raise both weights simultaneously and touch each shoulder with the weights. Repeat this exercise ten times every day and I guarantee results. Plus the strappy dresses will jump out of the closet.

For triceps, you need a bench or something flat and level. Check the photo. Then your arm swings like a pendulum. The repetition is ten times on each side. Is it too much? You are the one who wants muscles remember? And we are not even half way there.

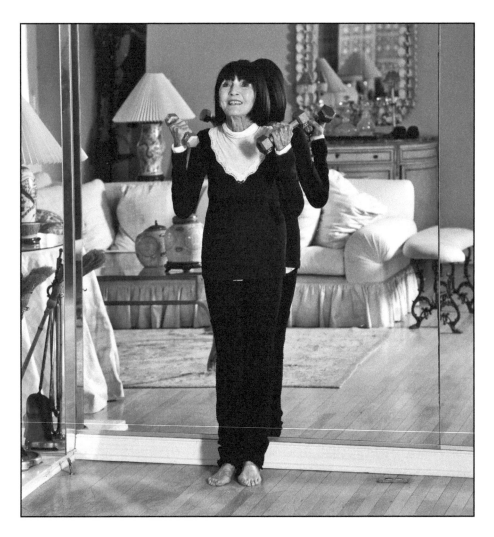

TIP #19 IMPERFECTIONS/INJURIES

Imperfections are part of your journey, and the other part is rising above the imperfections and dealing with them. **You cannot allow these nasty monsters to rule your life. You have to work with them, not against them.** I'm talking about arthritis, stenosis of the spine, rotator cuff, loose cartilage not only in knees, but also in the shoulders.

Actually arthritis responds well to activity and if you give in to this imperfection it will only get worse.

I have all these but (and it's a biggy), but I practice yoga. I took my first yoga class at 85 years, so age is not a factor. Arthritis is a given at any age not just 50 or 60.

Therapy is a big word and a given, and yoga, swimming, weights, and almost anything that keeps your joints and tendons and even your brain moving they are all a given. Not only a given but in my candid opinion one cannot live – I mean really live without any one of these vital activities.

So listen to me, I have spinal stenosis an abundance of arthritis and I practice yoga every day, dance tango every other day, and jump rope every day. And all my joints and muscles say thanks.

Maybe jump rope isn't going to be part of your daily routine but certainly you can do my 22 tips and maybe take a yoga class. Good idea-no?

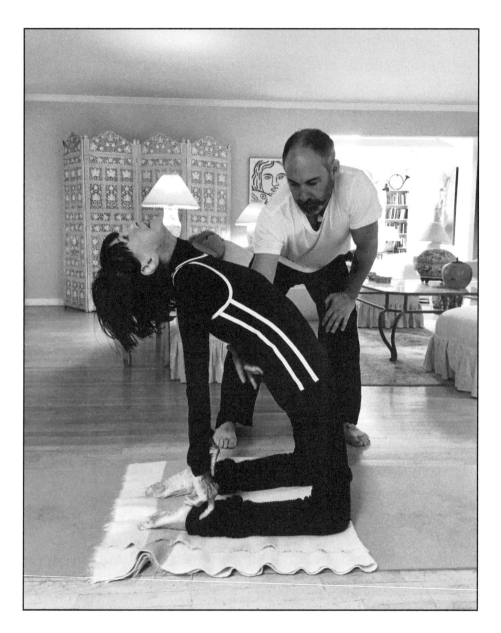

With Anthony Benenati,
my best friend and yoga mentor.

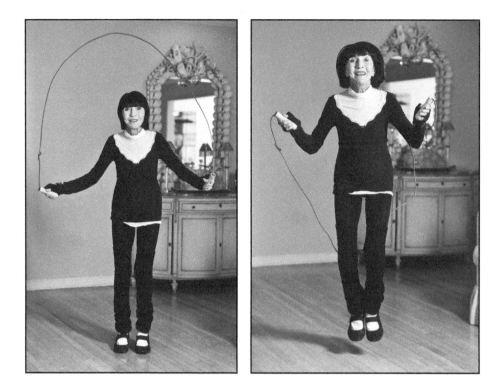

Tip #20 Jump Rope & Priorities

Every one of these exercises and poses I have written about and photographed are my daily routine plus a whole bunch more. **Only after you have mastered these nineteen, are you ready for my favorite – jump rope –** don't let it scare you.

Jump rope is great for your heart, your stamina, your feet, knees, and so many other things including joy. Just buy a rope and hang it some where so it's a reminder of things to come – like the pose **Peacock** [photo next page] This pose is a **priority** in my daily routine or I'll lose it, **And I want you to feel the same way about these 22 physical tips. They are all your priority for feeling**

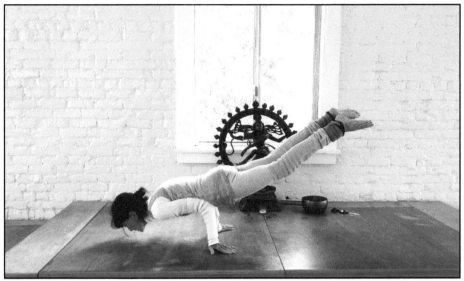

better. It's all about you. So loving yourself a little can go a long way.

Wanting to feel and look good is the issue, not age. 96 is no longer considered old, it's what you do at 96. Practice is never perfect, but then nothing is perfect. Building and facing the challenge is simply the right step, and taking action is the step toward success. Your desire to do something can outweigh your fear.

So enjoy the thought of what's possible, and go for it.

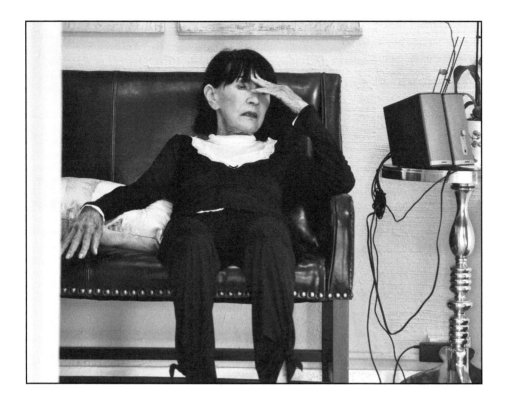

TIP #21 SICK

If by some chance you are sick, sit back and look at yourself and maybe you can see something that can help the problem... even solve the problem.

Relax completely. Have some words of wisdom with your body. Sometimes you have to give in. I didn't say give up – two different things.

When you give in, you let go. Letting go is very difficult for most people. It means opening up and exposing yourself. If you can do that comfortably it means at some time you decided to like yourself. When that happens, it's real and magical at the same time.

When you find that you like yourself, your feeling for everyone else will change, and you will look at the world around you with different eyes.

Making A Game Out Of Pain

Part of living is dealing with and overcoming the parts of one's body that start to give out. Like when one starts to face some areas of pain like arthritis, arteriosclerosis and loss of energy.

To continue a fulfilling life, one has to learn how to manage pain and to overcome and not slow down. THAT'S DIFFICULT. It takes lots of doing, not giving up, making a friend within yourself. *Did you know it's possible to make a friend within your own body. I'm talking about pain.*

Say you have pain that cannot be cured. It's living with you 24 hours a day. SOOOOO that pain becomes part of your body, part of your life. You learn to live with it. **Just as living is a learning process from your first breath of air, learning to live with pain is that same wonderful learning process. You learn to make friends with pain.** It becomes exactly the same as the pain when you stretch beyond your comfort zone, only it's not temporary, it's something you learn to manage and even something you can learn to like.

When I do a split on both left and right side I feel a real pull of muscles beyond my comfort zone. If I had to live 24 hours with that extension of muscle on the inside

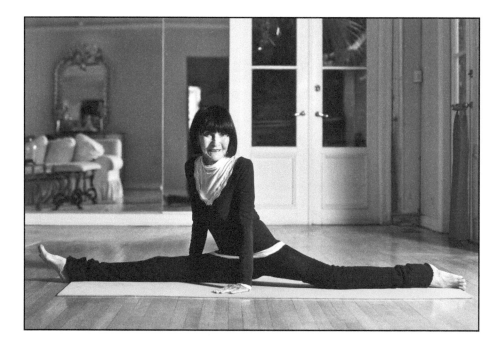

of my legs, I guess I would eventually make friends with that feeling and do no more complaining. **Complaining is a waste of energy and only encourages more pain.**

Who said this game is easy? The great challenge is keeping alive and growing as much as you can and then letting the chips fall where they may.

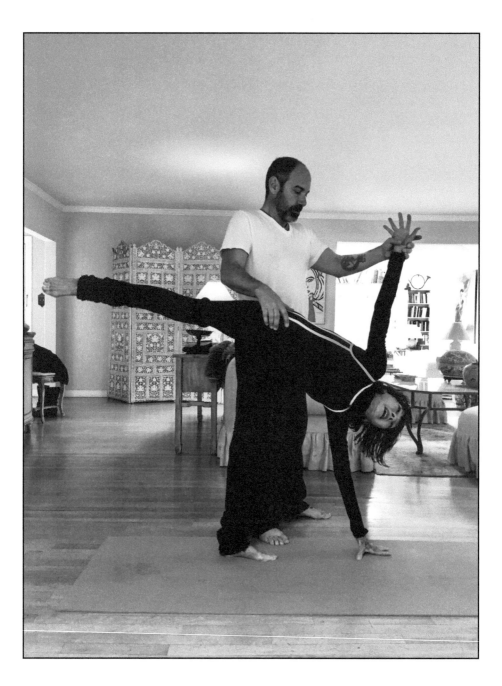

*Learning the Half Moon pose with Anthony Benenati,
my best friend and yoga mentor.*

Tip #22 – Why I'm still here

A gift to you.

I'm going to tell you in simple language how you can get to 96 in one word: **GIVE.**

I say give, and when I say GIVE, I will explain what that word means. It means GIVE TO YOUR BODY. **Your body needs this gift. It gives strength, stamina, and joy to you both.**

This means accept every challenge with activity, then take action.

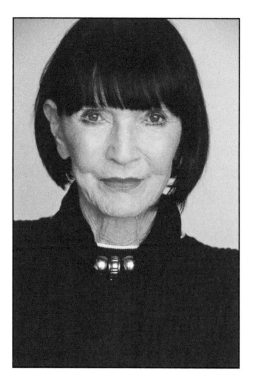

This means my 22 tips. *THIS MEANS MY 22 TIPS EACH DAY.*

Give your body time, love and knowledge. By knowledge I mean open up, listen, and be ready to face your body's needs. You don't realize it, but your body needs 24 hours of attention.

It's absolutely your best friend. It's completely truthful. It tells no lies.

You both need to indulge in conversation and pay attention.

Yes it's work, work, work. And this work pays off in millions of good healthy bones, muscles, and cells.

Please don't only **listen** to me. **Do something for yourself.**

There is only one reason to be here, and that's to be part of the universe. And the only way to be part of the universe is to be as creative as one possibly can. Doing is only half of it. Creating is the other half. So everything I do gives me the chance to breathe and live. It's giving to life, then life responds and you receive, and receive, and receive.

So what's it like to be 96?
Living 96 years can be
Years of happiness
Years of challenge
Years of learning
Years of understanding
and above all
Years of love

So you really want to know what it's like to be 96? Well there are moments great and small, perfect and not so perfect But I'm still here. *Hello 96.*

Freedom
Escape is not freedom
Presence is freedom

Freedom is a word that defies analyzation completely.

A word that ignites my desire to write what it means to me, and above all else lights a fire in my entire being.

"What gives us freedom?" and *"What freedom gives us?"* That's what its about. It's totally complex and totally fascinating.

Knowledge gives us freedom
Freedom gives us creativity
Physical strength gives us freedom
Fear kills freedom
Freedom gives us improvisation
Improvisation gives us freedom
Silence is freedom
Freedom is demanding
Multifaceted

All these things allow us to taste freedom, but being present is how we know freedom.

I can't think of a better way to experience and know freedom than our tip #11 Child pose. Your minutes in Child pose will open the doors to being present. *And being present is freedom.*

Moving and breathing are the greatest gift to man. But being present and knowing freedom is the next greatest gift.

Ode To Anthony Benenati

If only I could inspire the world not to give up
or give in.
There's always a way, an avenue, a possible process to heal,
to grow, and to listen.
It's not even complicated.
The simpler, the better.

I was told by knowledgeable doctors
I could never practice yoga again.
To me that was a death wish.
I toyed with that devastating idea for two months
feeling worse each day,
losing confidence, losing strength.
Where had that person called ME gone?
Even the energy that was *always there*
was slipping away.
Then the real ME awakened to an idea. Talk to, listen to that
person with whom you had seven years of living a complete,
healthy, constant active life of daily yoga practice
which had been totally cut off.
That person, my yoga mentor, generously gave me forty-five
minutes of his incredible knowledge.
My body not only responded, but absorbed
with such intensity that I could feel an amazing change
not only in body but in mind.
I knew then within forty-five minutes that yoga practice
had returned in full force and that I would always
do yoga to live and live to do yoga.

Spinal stenosis, arthritis, and osteoporosis
need not be the end of an active life.

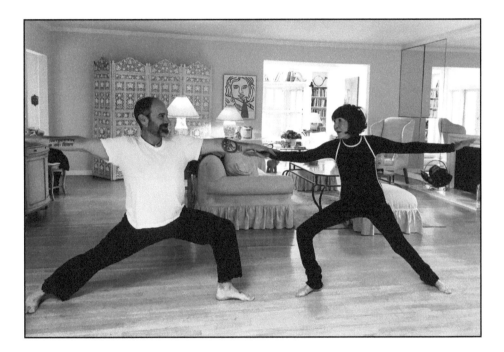

*Life is a discovery
and each day is an awakening.
Be present and taste freedom.
It's never too late.*

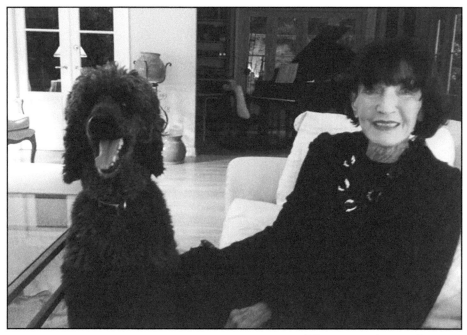

P.S.

Now that you've spent some time on yoga poses, stretches, and my exercises, how about spending the day with me?

Starting with *Good Morning, Good Morning.*

First, I have to walk Nicko (my poodle).

Then a unique and unusual **breakfast** starting with an eight ounce glass of water. Some espresso coffee, toast with butter-peanut butter, and top that with a thinly sliced banana.

This keeps me happy until lunch. **Lunch** is a chicken sandwich on whatever bread you prefer, plus lots of mayonnaise and lettuce. With juice of your choice and more water. During the pm, yogurt and apple sauce to hold me until dinner.

Dinner is Mediterranean diet. Sometimes more chicken, but veggies, salad with olive oil, lemon, Dijon mustard and garlic dressing.

If you're out to gain weight, it's lots of *Haagen-Daz* ice cream.

Here's a neat recipe for veggies:
one package of raw baby spinach
large fry pan
olive oil 2 tbs
shaved almonds
garlic – chopped
salt

Place spinach, garlic, almonds in the large frying pan with heated oil, no water. Stir-fry spinach almonds and garlic until spinach is soft and cooked. Add salt to taste.

Place all this in whatever electric mixer you use. Should be creamed. Now add 2 tablespoons plain yogurt, mix thoroughly, and have the taste thrill of your life. Almonds should be crunchy.

I also like mashed potatoes or baked potato, and sautéed chicken, plus a salad. I love my creamed spinach on the baked potato.

This dinner is so light and tasty. I can eat this every night. But I'm definitely not normal.

If your aim is to lose weight cut out the butter. Don't forget to drink water. It's your life, plus breathing, and my tips.

Bon Appetite

See you tomorrow.

Life is a discovery
Each day is an awakening
AND IT'S NEVER EVER TOO LATE

EPILOGUE

Eight men and three women are responsible for these stories. I dedicate this journey of 96 years to:

My mother **Gladys Gehrig**, without whom there would be no dancer, fashion designer, musician, or writer.

Jose Fernandez, who taught and inspired me to *be* and perform classic Spanish dance.

Agnes DeMille, who gave me and the world four hit Broadway shows.

Jerry Robbins and *High Button Shoes,* without whom I wouldn't have met **Donnie Weissmuller** who made me laugh and dance to exciting choreography.

Alan Sues, my first husband, who gave me the ability and confidence to be funny and sing.

Norman Pincus, my second husband, who backed and encouraged me 100% to be a successful fashion designer.

Joyce Collins, a singer and musician who freed me to write songs and tangos.

Gudni Gunnarson, creator of Rope Yoga and a most valued friend in my life.

Felix Chavez, who gave me my first tango lesson and a life and challenge beyond my imagination.

Anthony Benenati my first and only yoga teacher, friend, and mentor.

Marcos Questas, who gave me confidence and the ability to follow his amazing lead. And perhaps the reality of a continuing journey for who knows how long.

I would not be who I am today were it not for the love inspiration and guidance of these amazing men and women.

Thank you.

Once in a while I think of the reality of the number 96 and I spread my wings.

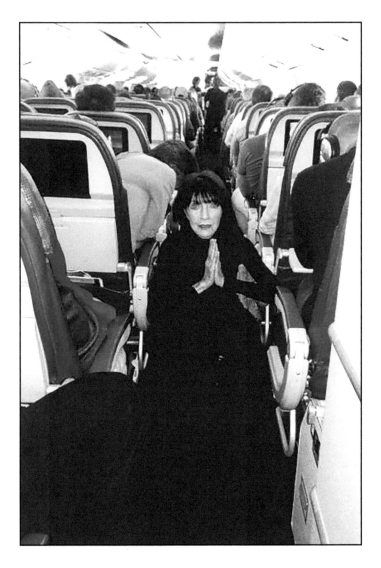

*There's a yoga studio on every L.A. corner,
but only one on this 747. Yoga is my way of
life on the ground and in the air.*

Moments to share...

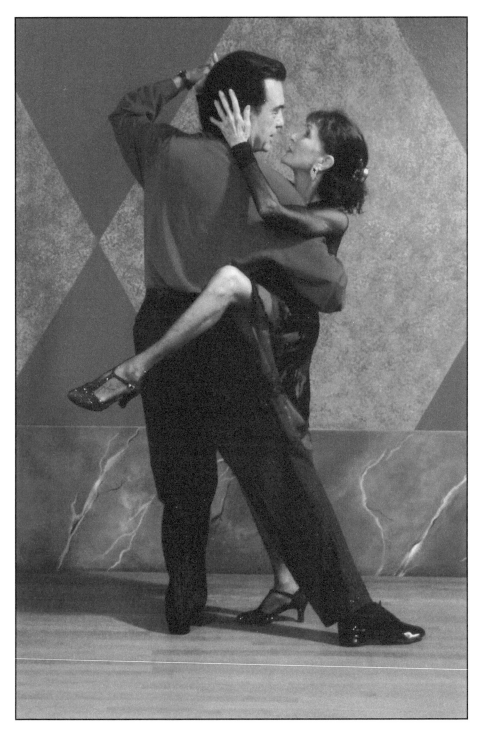

Felix Chavez (photographer unknown)

MY TANGO SONG

I've been learning the tango
it seems forever
so many things to learn and remember
don't use your brain
use your feet

soften your arms
and feel the beat

learn how to follow
will I ever
just give in, it's now or never

black and blue shins
painful toes
why cant I do this difficult pose

guess I'll just write good prose

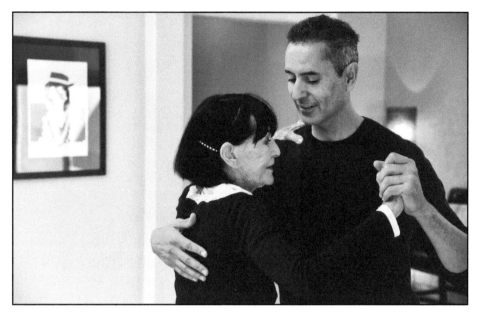

Marcos Questas is the teacher who finally taught me to follow.
(photo by Adam Sheridan-Taylor)

If only I could follow

If only I could follow like I should
Doin' a crusada would be good
A boleo would be better
Than an ocho double header
An a goncho yo no puedo
Because I'm so affredo
If only I could follow like I should
That would be oh so good

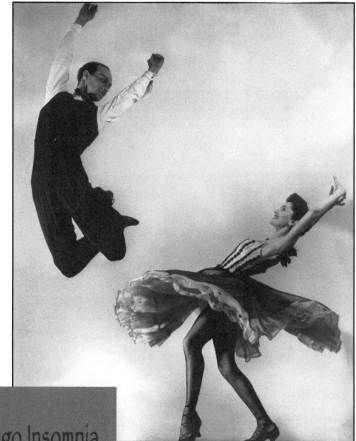

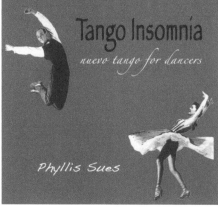

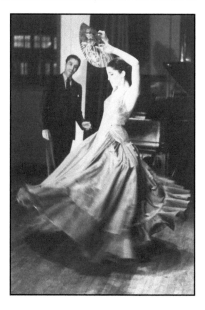

*Top: Donnie Weissmuller and I
(1949)
Left: My Tango CD (2008)
Right: Jose Fernandez and I
(1941)
(photographers unknown)*

79

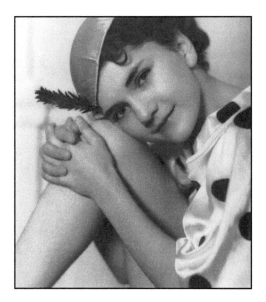

Left: age ten

*Below: about age
twenty-five*

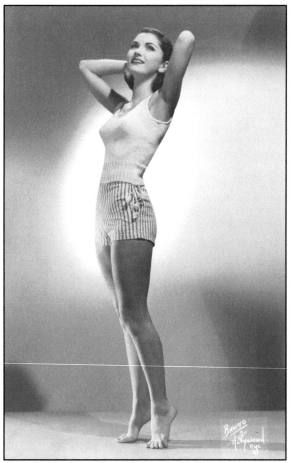

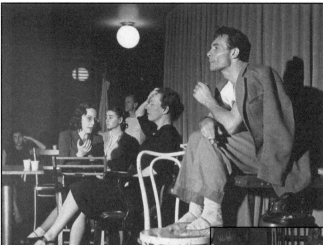

*In rehearsal for **Brigadoon**
on Broadway.
Above: Agnes DeMille and
James Mitchell,
Right: James Mitchell and
Lidija Franklin
(photographers unknown)*

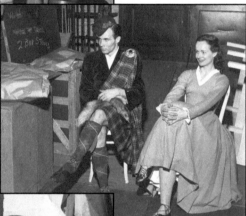

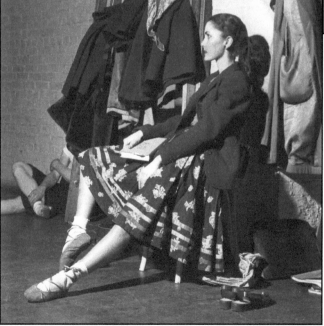

*Me backstage
on break during
rehearsals at the
Ziegfield Theater
for **Brigadoon**
(photographer
unknown)*

Playing Monopoly with the stars of **Bloomer Girl** *on Broadway (photographer unknown)*

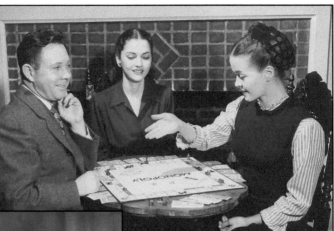

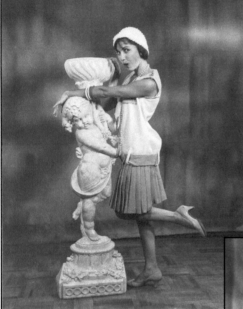

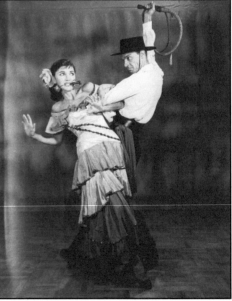

Above: **The Boyfriend**
Right: **Can Can** *with Donnie Weissmuller*
Both productions at Sacramento Music Circus 1960 (photographer unknown)

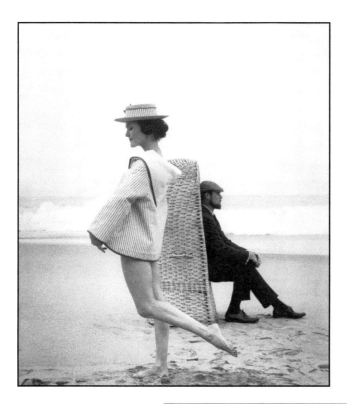

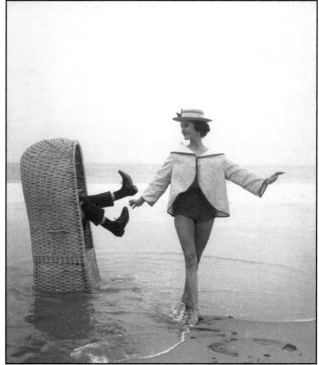

Fun on Santa Monica Beach with Stephen Ferry-Fashions by Phyllis (photos by Joyce Rainboldt)

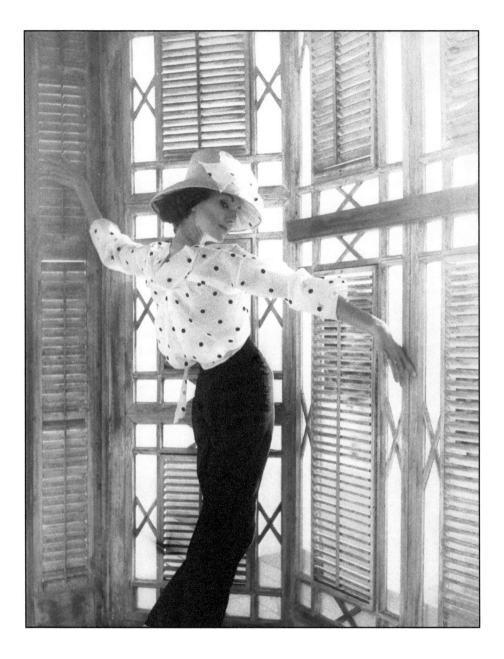

*Above: Alan Sues was also a wonderful photographer. He and I
would set up photo shoots for which I would create the fashions.
(Right - photo by Joyce Rainboldt)*

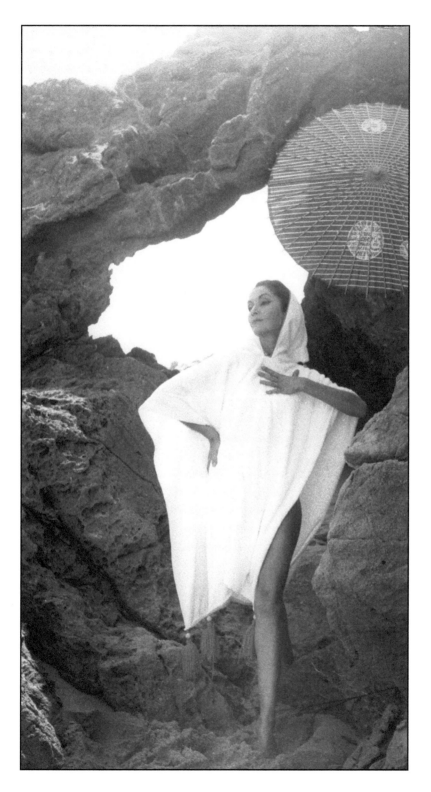

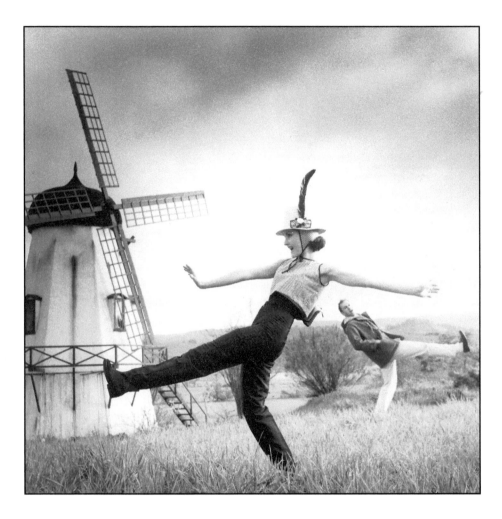

Alan and I playing on camera.
(photo by Joyce Rainboldt)

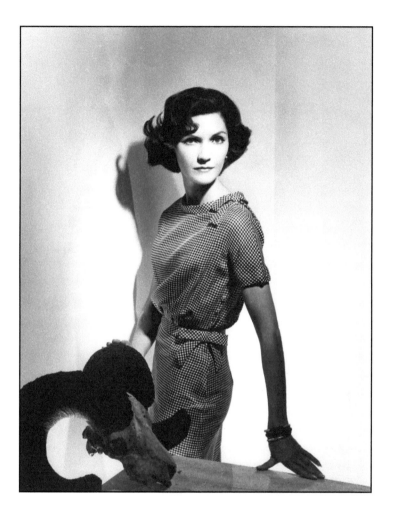

Photography by Edward Carroll

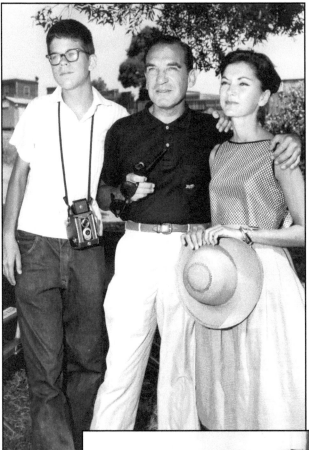

With my second husband, Norman, and my step-son, Charles.

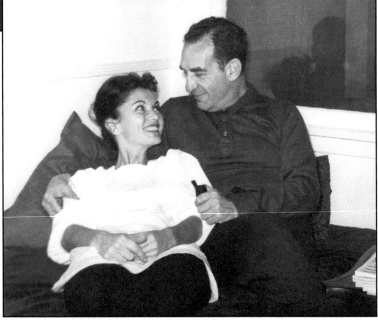

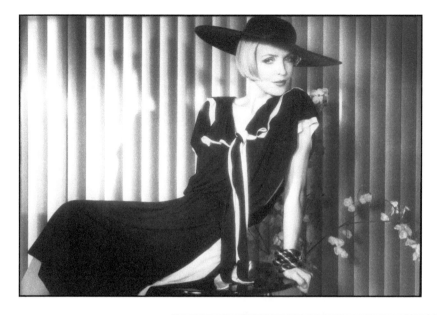

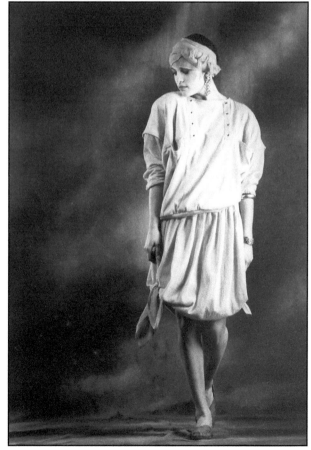

Norman helped me to establish my career as a fashion designer. Two models wearing my designs. (photographers unknown)

I tried skydiving for my 90th birthday. Then went back a second time.

New experiences are important!

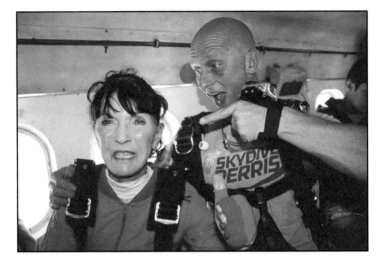

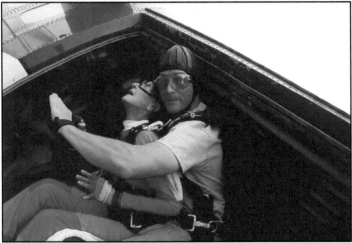

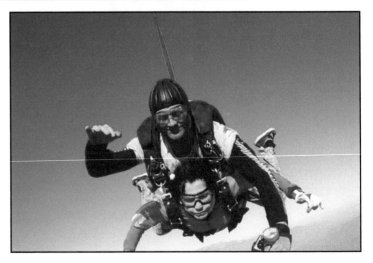

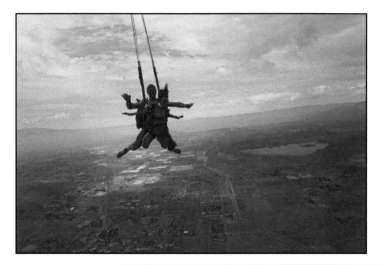

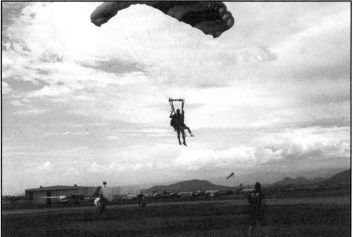

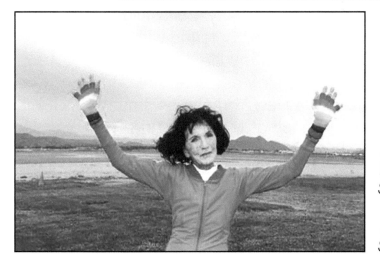

Photo credit:
Kris Peterson
Skydive Perris
Phyllis with
Simeon Lott/
Skydive Perris

Some of my Blogs from
the *Huffington Post*

NYC vs. LA
12/13/2013

Being born is one thing. Being born in NYC in 1923 is the best thing! That year has colored my entire life. To be a part of the Broadway scene in 1944, and to dance in the *Shubert Theater,* and walk through stage door 6, nights and matinées. That was living!

Sardi's across the street and the *Astor Hotel* on the corner. The show was *Bloomer Girl* with Celeste Holm. Agnes DeMille choreography, Harold Arlen music with Yip Harburg lyrics.

Those were Broadway's golden years! No repeats, all originals. You could sense the rumble of McCarthyism and the smell of the black list. Within the company of *Bloomer Girl,* there were many political activists. Not me, I was a dancer's dancer, bursting with energy. I lived for dance and dance was my life. Fast-forward to 1956 and Los Angeles. The air was breathable, the sky was blue. The climate to a New Yorker was amazing, but the culture and energy was not yet happening. That was yet to come.

New York is a city of speed and energy. Even if you didn't make it, you thought you were making it! No one walks in New York, they run. But, the culture on a scale of 10, was a 10 and still is. The theater page in the *NY Times* is multiple pages. Don't forget that coffee, and the subway was a nickel.

Los Angeles is not a city of speed. It's a slow moving city. It was years before I found my place in LA. This is a city for self-starters. One doesn't get the push and sense of energy needed to succeed. The difference in LA between 1956 and 2013 culturally and creatively, can knock your socks off! The #1 symphony in the world, first-class opera and the jazz scene is percolating.

And that leads me to the fashion scene in the 60s. LA was considered a beachwear city. NY was the capitol of fashion in the USA, but in the 70s there was a young fashion group of which I was a major part and that group, plus the entire LA fashion scene, escalated into a very sophisticated competitive industry that still exists.

Entering the fashion scene now in 2013 takes youthful fearlessness, naïveté, and beaucoup bucks. My exit came after 22 years and was timely. I loved every minute of those 22 years and I'm loving all the years that have followed. Even Los Angeles! This is where I dance, make music, face challenges (sky dive) and if I may be so bold, know and like who I am. That's taken a few years, but it's not the number. It's simply the time. It's never too late. It's always the beginning.

How Tango Lessons Changed This 91-Year-Old's Life
08/28/2014

Tango, salsa, samba, rumba, bolero. All the Latin dances, bring crowds to the dance floor. But one stands apart, with star quality. TANGO! Just the name alone has a sound different from all the rest. And the music! The music! The music, wow! Brings emotion, that no other can compare. What is it about tango that makes your heart beat faster? Makes your body linger close to your partner. You feel unexplainable sensations, because you and your partner have become one. And yet at that same moment, you have not lost self.

That is the secret and the beauty, when two dancers become one. When tango is danced in this magical way, it looks so simple. But by no means is tango simple. Once you're hooked on tango, you will work to perfect this dance for the rest of your life and you will never attain that perfection.

Tango is a life long marriage. Just the terminology of each move has magic. *Boleo, ocho, cruzada, gancho* and to master these moves smoothly and with power, takes a lifetime. Argentineans are born dancing tango. Learning and imitating, their grandparents and parents. They grow up with that gorgeous music. That music that demands one's complete attention, not to miss a beat. The rhythm that is so unexpected. The beat that changes constantly and requires a good ear.

As my first tango teacher, Felix Chavez says, *"You dance in the music, not to the music."*

My first tango lesson was a disaster, even though my training has been ballet and modern. I froze from fear, and I would not follow my partner. There are some who are natural followers, but that was not to be my good fortune. I started six years ago at age 85. I'm 91 and I'm still desperately trying to achieve that attainable and natural moment of feeling one, with my partner and teacher, Marcos Questas, a superb professor of tango, who has the great quality of humor and kindness, beyond the norm.

Tango is the cure-all and end-all of depression. It stimulates energy, emotion, balance and the curious thing called life. There is no age limit. Tango brings joy and physical ability, you didn't know you had. Just like I had no idea, I could compose six tangos and put together a successful CD, *Tango Insomnia* with six fabulous musicians.

So, you see the inspiration came from that Argentine music. Just writing about it makes my body undulate. So, spend an evening at a Milonga. Starting with a tango class and then dance the night away. What's more important; the price is right. The place to go is called a Milonga. Google, *Milonga* and you will discover Milongas everywhere, not only in L.A., but every city in the U.S.A., and every city in Europe.

So, no excuse not to experiment! You too will be inspired to dance to that beautiful Argentine tango music. You will love it, and your body will love it, and your partner will love you! How can you resist?

It's never, never too late! One day you will believe me. When that happens, that will be the best day of your life. Dance to the rhythm of the tango and live.

Happy New Year! Oh Yeah?
01/09/2016

Happy New Year! Will it be or won't it be? That's the million-dollar unanswerable question. Looking at what we have right now, I wish I could feel optimistic. In my personal life, I love what I do, what I have, and what I have had. There is fear and questioning and loss of confidence in our leadership. Loss of strength and loss of dynamic guidance. The hope is that the next chosen one will take the reins and lead this wonderful country in a positive and healthy direction. And my biggest and desperate wish is that, that leader will be someone with compassion for a country who has honesty and integrity. A country that has arrived partially to accepting all colors — and not only all colors, but all people from all countries. A country that honors freedom of speech, thoughts and religion. I want to live and die here. I want to embrace and love this country and let 2016 be a good one.

The word Happy regarding this New Year in each of us in my candid opinion does not ring with great hope. Peace is a better word and so a better expression would be "let's have a peaceful new year" and a loving, compassionate one and, yes, one free of fear. Fear breeds disaster, but being aware and truthful and completely present encourages confidence in each of us and the whole world will take notice and respond. Is that too optimistic? Maybe, but it's a step in a positive direction for the new year. I refuse to think and behave in a negative way. It does not produce a healthy mind and body.

So let's talk about celebration, not just once a year,

but a celebration each day we wake up to a country at peace — to a world at peace and to a day we can breathe clean air, see the sun in the morning, the moon and stars at night and feel the raindrops on our cheeks, and a day free of cancer.

Life doesn't move rapidly. It grows and we grow with it. If you really want something to celebrate try this scenario.

Celebrate;
Waking up.
Being born.
Being healthy, mentally and physically.
Liking what you do.
Who you are.
And being aware of every waking moment.

And most of all celebrate being alive and living on this planet.

So let's celebrate the possibility of living a healthy, peaceful life in this universe and Mars too. So let the stars shine and give thanks for another year.

Let 2016 be a happy one.

Effects and Effects
03/31/2016

Just came back from the dentist and the removal of a tooth and root and four stitches after which the dentist said, *"here, fill this prescription, it's an antibiotic"* and my immediate reaction was, *"Uh-uh! Can't take it, really bad side effects."* Those two words "side effects" stuck in my brain and started it dancing. Have you any idea of how many side effects we live with and never think about?

Here are just a few:

The side effects of eating.
The side effects of smoking.
The side effects of marriage.
The side effects of divorce.
The side effects of friendships.
The side effects of lies.
And let's not forget politics.
And there are many more.

But for me the best side effect of living 93 years is feeling good, liking who I am and loving this incredible long journey. There is no future and no past. So just "being" is a pretty good side effect of living. So let's just think about the good side effects of living, starting with that guy you have lived with all your life, your body. That guy who talks to you constantly. That guy who gives you everything to live for, your body, and the good side effects that come when you respond. Mentally and physically with no excuses, no minuses. No hesitation. Now you will be astonished at all the good side effects. It's called getting up out of that chair and into the God-given air we all take for granted. Just as we all take for granted our amazing machine that wants and demands to be used and loved. Ninety-three is only a number, but a beautiful number when experienced with love, energy and trust.

There's a trophy to be had, but it doesn't come without work and — surprisingly enough — joy. So we need desperately to like ourselves. Then and only then can we like what we do. Then and only then can living have good side effects.

Nothing is perfect, but it can always be better. Don't get me wrong, I love side effects, good and bad. They teach us and we learn from them. We can't live without them. We should listen and respond to them just as we should listen and respond to our amazing first instrument — our body.

I like my life that should be a given for everyone, but one has to be open to all of its wonders that want to be ignited. It's possible to find the embers and light the flame of creativity. By creativity I mean find the outlet that brings you joy and a rich life. Part of the side effect is longevity and if we accept the challenge, it can be good longevity. Listening to my first instrument is the best and only way to enjoy the journey.

Birthdays are meaningless if you're living each and every minute in the moment. That's living in the present. So let's open the gates and welcome all the side effects. Good and bad. Can't live without them.

What I've Learned About Birthdays After 93 Years
04/01/2016

I just decided I'm not having one.

It's enough to know I was born April 4, 1923, so Monday, April 4, 2016 will be the usual. Another expected and unexpected day in my life. Waking at 6 a.m. and 45 minutes of yoga stretches and poses. My usual breakfast: oatmeal, honey, cinnamon, walnuts (for the brain) protein powder (for the joints) and espresso (for the boost).

Now I'm ready for yoga class with yoga master Anthony Benenati. Now I'm ready for a short nap. Then 12 minutes on the bike and now I'm ready for the love of my life, TANGO, with the one and only Marcos Questas, friend, teacher, and unbeatable tango dancer.

Now I'm completely energized — body and brain — and I'm not sure who I am much less what day it is. So much for this birthday. There is no complaint coming. I have lived 93 years with no stop sign in sight. Nothing wrong with that scenario.

If I'm going to celebrate, it's going to be a celebration of waking each day with the same energy and love for living. Now, that's worth celebrating, but I'm not going to bore you with the history of my life, which has been totally wonderful and unexpected and with a little luck will continue. It doesn't have to be today, it's every day.

Birthdays are great at 20 and iffy at 50 and at 70 well, that's up to you and your body and what to do with the rest of your life. Got to invent, got to think positive, and if you haven't already listened to your body, now's the time to listen and respond. Now's the time to move.

Yoga, tennis, dance, walk and run, if you still can. Try something new; piano, guitar, learn a foreign language. You just might surprise yourself and discover a new career. I've had four and could be a fifth just waiting. Just keep saying, *"Yes, yes, yes, I love this life."* And I like me too, which means I like you too, so if the number means just a number, *"go for it."* For me, it will always be just a number, which might just continue to be another and another and another.

So, as time marches on and so do birthdays, there are changes in our attitude between one another and how we handle these changes. Personally, I find recently when an argument develops instead of getting all fired up, I tend to step back and soften. This is new for me and I like it.

It's enjoying the cool feeling of being cool, which comes from watching and being on the outside rather than being in the middle of a conversation gone sour. It's being completely present — a wonderful place to be and very difficult to achieve.

So closing with that powerful word PRESENT, I want to wish and say to all of you, whatever number you chose and whatever day you celebrate happy birthday, face every challenge with joy, energy, love, the possibility and the knowledge that life and birthdays will continue. But not least, let's all celebrate a world at peace.

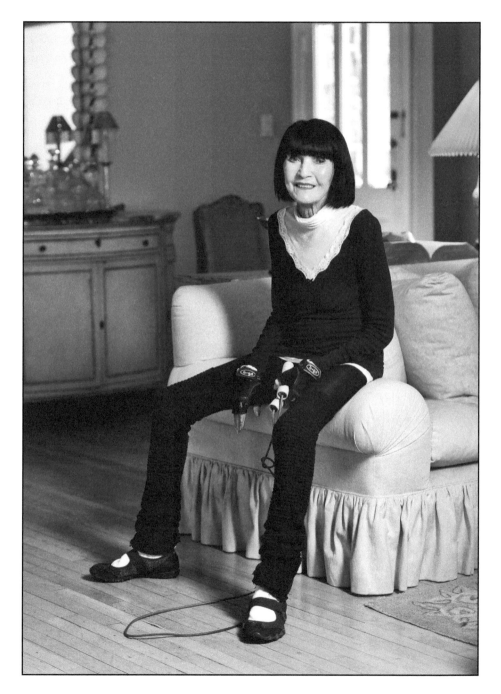

Blue Tuesday And The Waiting Game
11/29/2016

I say Blue Tuesday not because it's the Democrats insignia on the map but because it's the saddest day for America. The electoral vote escapes me since the popular vote is the honest most realistic vote because it's my vote, your vote and every one's vote — so why do we bother to go through all this madness? Yes this undemocratic election system became the Electoral College over 200 years ago. At that time it was purely a political deal and now it's still a political deal. In the 1800s, it was rigged for Republicans and still is. Even now our two senators from San Francisco are introducing a bill to kill the electoral college — good luck to them. In 2000, Al Gore got the popular vote and lost the electoral vote and now we are faced with a completely inadequate president elect, who neither understands this democracy nor has the expertise to lead this country. A disaster for America and all its citizens who make America what it is. And I'm feeling so very helpless as not a joiner, not a protester — but just an ordinary citizen loving my country and hoping that a miracle will happen. But as optimistic as I am, it's not realistic to say let's just wait and see. Wait and see a massive disaster. We have yet to hear one word of inspiration that's feasible and financially possible and would take again, expertise to accomplish in our current situation. I'm not saying either nominee is perfect but experience, knowledge and in this case world knowledge would be helpful to put it gently.

As a country that has greatness and understands the importance and salvation of dealing with a world of so many different countries that are dependent on one another. I'm feeling our present president elect is completely surreal and has neither the experience nor the expertise to work with not only our government, but all governments. Out of 300 million people living in this country, well I'm not going to even finish this sentence. Oh my God, just the thought of four years with this president elect with his sunshine yellow hair gives me chills. And how is this president elect going to communicate with the women in his Cabinet, who he has so demonized? Don't tell me to be patient and wait and see. I don't see light at the end of this tunnel — I see dark and chaos.

And what about climate change, which is up for grabs or not even at all, which in every way has been proven scientifically for years to be the effect of human behavior. Will we see all the work that has been done by world powers smashed because one person with extreme power and no expertise refuses to believe the proven truth?

It's a wonderful country that has chosen this man to lead America. Shame on us! During the months of campaigning my thoughts were *"this is a comedy, I wish it were just a farce"* and I would wake up tomorrow and the play is over. But instead I wake up every morning with a deadly feeling that this is reality and I can't wait to practice yoga, where for one hour I will be connected to the universe and not this comedy of errors.

But no matter where this election takes us — let's keep pushing and believing. We live in a true democracy and a really true blue America and a country where freedom isn't just for a few, but every living American of every color, every gender and every race.

Please let this be a given, not just a hope.

MARRIAGE / WHY

I've been married twice both times in a church. Once in New York City, once in Las Vegas. Both included legal documents that proved I was really married. But, the other day I needed something in my file where I keep important documents and those marriage documents were not to be found. Both Alan and Norman, my first and second husbands, have long since left this planet. So, since I can't prove I was married both times does that mean I was never married? And is that really important?

I'm 93 going on 94 in 1 month. Maybe it would be important if I were an immigrant under this unfortunate administration but since I was born in the U.S.A. and have a passport (incidentally it needs to be renewed) I probably won"t be deported.

So marriage is not a priority at least in my current life. I'm often asked if I had the opportunity would I consider marriage again? *"You must be kidding – WHY?"*

Life is a constant challenge and living single is a difficult challenge (though a good one), but marriage is and I have to say it THE MOST DIFFICULT CHALLENGE.

Living with and not married to, was the very best relationship in my life and would have been the longest in my life had it not been for the unbeatable cancer. So if it's the love of your life no matter how you decide to go it, marriage or no marriage, it's worth it.

During those twelve years we talked about getting

married – maybe on a tennis court.

We both played tennis badly, during our time on the court we sounded like John McEnroe on his worst day. Why we ever played together has always puzzled me. Guess that's why we never got married on or off the tennis court. What we had was understanding, giving, and unconditional love. If you have all three of these the purpose of marriage is obsolete.

Perhaps you were brought up knowing you would find Mr. Right and the gown, the bridesmaids, and the expected elaborate show that was and is not uncommon to this day.

Remember this writer is 93 which we all know is simply a number in reality. I have no idea what age I am. I just know the journey has been rewarding, always creative, and above all challenging. The most challenging years were both marriages. The second marriage was like falling off a building. He saved me and I never questioned or even hesitated. If I had to do it all over again I would probably do exactly the same.

It takes years to give birth to, recognize and appreciate wisdom. I'm still working on it. So being candid and honest, I've lived with someone three times in my life and each one was (to say the least) unusual, fulfilling, loving and worth all the ups and downs, and lots of both.

So whatever you choose let it be with love. Loving someone takes priority over every word you've just read.

But I'm not through yet.

Getting married for monetary reasons or convenience or any other thing without love is a loser, you'll never make it. Maybe you'll stay hitched, but the joy and living a life of quality will never happen.

A part of a relationship that cannot be ignored is the physicality and chemistry that goes with a new found relationship – sometimes lasting but in most cases not the case. What's needed here is a meeting of the minds.

I've seen couples who have never had a physical attraction but mentally they were one person. So many qualities spell a lasting relationship.

Best that you know who you are, respect who you are, and recognize these qualities in that chosen person.

A solo life only works if you have found your métier, and are good at it. At this time in my life I'm open to new adventures and love the ones I'm living with. The knowledge that anything is possible excites me.

This philosophy didn't come to life in my life until my 70s when music became an integral part of every part of me. Not out of desperation, but out of acceptance and the challenges in front of me. Listening to your body and your mind – *both of which are your only and best friends in my eyes* – is the best marriage around.

I'll buy that.

This is a marriage of reality and love.

What a beautiful combination.

My best time with the person I love is bed time. I don't mean sex time. Just being close physically, emotionally and mentally, that's the time to relate deeply. No hangups. Just awareness of each other's wondrous giving and accepting qualities.

To have this kind of relationship is to have everything possible.

Go for it, accept it. It's the winning ticket.

Are you listening?

Thoughts Of An Aspiring Writer
11/20/2015

Why do I write? Where does it come from? I would like to write like I talk. Thank goodness, I write better than I talk because when I talk I can't always find the words at that exact moment. Whereas when I write, I always find the words because I have time. When I read what I have written I'm smitten with amazement. How did I create that sentence? When I read one of my blogs at that moment I say, *"I'm possibly a good writer"*, then I immediately say, *"who am I to say I'm even a writer?"* I like what I write and am surprised by its originality. Is that egotistical, self-centered? Who says I'm a good writer? Is it just *Huffington Post?* My friends say you should write a book about your life. My response is "How?" I need help to organize all the multitude of pages of autobiographical writing. Where do I begin? HELP!

When I write I never forget. When I speak I always forget. But there are four times in my life when the challenge of not forgetting and being totally present take hold and bring me to a wonderful place. They are in this order: writing, tango, cooking and yoga. If I could ask for the most difficult to accomplish, the most challenging, those four would be at the top of the list. Actually meditation and being present should be simultaneous. And for me the almost impossible to achieve. It's not a question of not being present, it's a question of insecurity and daring to doubt or daring to compliment or accepting the fact that perhaps just maybe you're not really all that bad.

Read the blogs. Don't they speak to you, tell you

something? No matter what you think and criticize, if you write with creativity and humor, there you go again thinking in pluses and minuses, positives and negatives. It's that, that makes us frail and strong and human. We think in dark and light and, as Gudni Gudnnarsson says, *"there is no dark, light dispels the dark."* I like that! We have to shine our light on the dark. Wow! That's good. I'm going to bed now and shine my light on my dreams, so that they will all be wonderful, full of beautiful performances like dancing, turning (no stopping), jumping (no descending). Dreams are the most important part of sleep, if only we could remember them.

When I'm quiet and truly listening ... that's when the present is a possibility and even a reality. And that's when writing presents itself in a creative way. I have to admit the creative moments are never when I'm at the computer. Those moments appear while I'm lying on my bed half sitting, half lying. Sometimes while I'm sleeping a phrase or an idea will wake me and I'm impelled to sit up and turn on the light, find the paper and pen and write. Damn, now I'm wide awake. If I wait until morning that fabulous thought will have escaped. I guess all writers have their idiosyncrasies or hang ups. So am I a writer? I constantly ask myself that question. My answer is in and out. Yes and no, but the challenge is always there facing me, daring me, exciting me, and driving me to put the pen on the paper and speak.

One more thought. Try being present while driving your car. You might remember how you got to where you're going. And if you can't remember how you got to where you were going, try cooking.

Auditions And The Unknown Ingredient
10/14/2015

I haven't auditioned in over 70 years, so doing an audition at this time in my life is not exactly the norm. Doing a simple audition with sides (that's a scene or scenes in a movie, TV show or commercial) is one thing, but performing as a *yenta* a gossipy Jewish lady with a heavy Yiddish accent is entirely another venue. Not entirely impossible, just challenging to say the least.

I auditioned for the first time at age 18 for a Broadway show **Pretty Penny**. Michael Kidd was the choreographer and George Kaufman was the director. Within the dance group there were maybe eight girl and eight boy dancers. Two became famous — Peter Gennaro, who was hearing impaired and practiced with headphones,

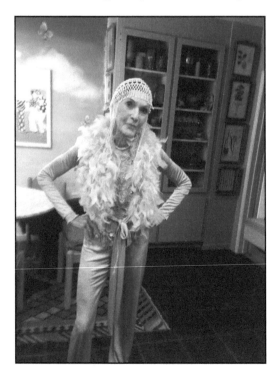

and Onna White, who became a successful choreographer and director. It was one of those shows that never made it to Broadway, but for all of us dancers, it was an introduction to *The Great White Way.*

Seventy-two years later, here in Tinsel Town L.A., the movie capital of the world, I am making an attempt to enter this crazy overcrowded overrated, star-studded business. I use the term *business* because when you say I'm in the *business* everyone knows you mean movies or TV.

A dance audition is one thing I'm familiar with, delighted with and nervous with. But, speaking lines? Yes, I'm also familiar with those, but it's been a while since the successful TV show **The Real McCoy's** during the 60s in which I said lines and had a one-shot part with Dick Crenna who knew I was a newcomer to this *"business"* and let me know that I was not to step on his lines — *"oops."*

At that time, I was dancing and performing on multiple variety shows like Dinah Shore, Andy Williams, etc. Now with my 92 years of wisdom and being totally fearless, I appeared at this audition as an older Jewish yenta speaking with a heavy Yiddish accent. Now that's a challenge for this *goy.* I hadn't a clue, but with guts and some anxiety I threw myself into this amazing experience, having fun and doing something foreign vocally and physically.

So, as I live a long and most unexpected life, which seems to be never-ending, there is light at the end of the tunnel. It took a dare for my first sky-dive, but no dare for the second and third coming up! And there was no audition for the trapeze or skydiving — just no fear and a big challenge. So in a way, doing a yenta and speaking with a Yiddish accent takes the same ingredients — plus a little innocence. One thing about dance auditions is that you know by the end of the audition if you are the chosen one out of 100 other dancers. In film it's a waiting game. And god only knows how many other contestants are vying for the same yenta.

But now in my enviable long life I'm quite calm. I guess because I loved performing that yenta and even have the nerve to say maybe my accent was OK. Did I look 70? I thought so, but that's my egotistical opinion. I didn't get a call back. So I'll never know. That's the unknown ingredient.

Every performer, be it on stage or in film or on the tennis court, wants to be the winner and the chosen one. I mention tennis because that was my most favorite game and only game of my life. So now auditions are simply another part of this incredible, unexplainable and wonderful journey. Do I get nervous? I certainly hope so. I would hate to lose that youthful emotion. No nerves, no performance.

This message would not be complete without a word of praise for the sunshine in my life. No matter how I feel — fatigued, in pain, or sick — yoga, will always be a part of my daily routine. Practice is the building block, the joy, and the wake-up call each and every day of my life. I live to do yoga, and I do yoga to live.

Phyllis Sues, a dedicated yogi.

Breathing And Being

How many days and nites ahead
Just breathing and being is enough
Well said

So reach for the sky and
Touch a star we'er together
To do or die

Give love and joy
to all things living
then this day will
be one of giving

Cherish this day
there will be another
It's never to late
to love each other

or did you forget?????

What will be it like when I'm 99?

What's it gonna be when I'm 99?
well, I'll give it a try
and I'll just be fine.
Will it be different?
Will I have time?
Will it be the same at 99?

Wake up every morning,
think I'm 29,
doin' 20 push-ups
and the world is mine.

My skin is thin
and they say I'm skinny,
but I don't care 'cause
I still can do the shimmy.

Doin' those push ups,
stand on my head.
Hey you guys
I ain't dead.

Don't stop now.
Your life can be a beautiful journey.